LCHF COOKBOOK

MAIN COURSE - 60+ Low-Carb, High-Fat Breakfast, Lunch, Dinner and Dessert Recipes

TABLE OF CONTENTS

BREAKFAST 7

PINEAPPLE PANCAKES 7

ALMOND PANCAKES 9

APPLE PANCAKES 11

STRAWBERRY PANCAKES 13

PEAR PANCAKES 15

GINGERBREAD MUFFINS 17

CHERRIES MUFFINS 19

BLUEBERRY MUFFINS 21

BERRIES MUFFINS 23

CHOCOLATE MUFFINS 25

RASPBERRIES MUFFINS 27

LETTUCE OMELETTE 29

ZUCCHINI OMELETTE 31

JICAMA OMELETTE 33

MUSHROOM OMELETTE 35

BASIL OMELETTE 37

HASH BROWN EGG NESTS 39

BREAKFAST BARS 41

MORNING GRANOLA 43

STREUSEL SCONES 45

LUNCH 47

PUMPKIN FRITATTA 47

SPINACH FRITATTA 49

KALE FRITATTA 51

SNOW PEAS FRITATTA 53

BROCCOLI FRITATTA 55

SALMON WITH HERB SAUCE 57

GLAZED PORK CHOPS 59

VEGGIES PIZZA 61

LIVER AND MASHED VEGETABLES 63

LEMON CHICKEN 65

CALIFORNIA SALAD 67

QUINOA SALAD 68

PANZANELLA SALAD 69

BASIL SALAD 70

TOMATO SALAD 71

POTATO SALAD 72

HAWAIIAN SALAD 73

COLESLAW 74

KALE SALAD 75

ICEBERG WEDGE SALAD 76

DINNER 77

SIMPLE PIZZA RECIPE 77

ZUCCHINI PIZZA 79

CAULIFLOWER RECIPE 80

BROCCOLI RECIPE 81

TOMATOES & HAM PIZZA 82

LEEK SOUP 84

ZUCCHINI SOUP 85

OKRA SOUP 88

RED BELL PEPPER SOUP 90

POTATO SOUP 92

SMOOTHIES 94

PINK SMOOTHIE 94

APPLE BANANA SMOOTHIE 95

CARDAMOM SMOOTHIE 96

VEGAN SMOOTHIE 97

BLACKBERRY SMOOTHIE 98

STRAWBERRY SMOOTHIE 99

MANGO SMOOTHIE 100

BANANA SMOOTHIE 101

SUMMER SMOOTHIE 102

DETOX SMOOTHIE 103

Copyright 2019 by Noah Jerris - All rights reserved.

This document is geared towards providing exact and reliable information in regards to the topic and issue covered. The publication is sold with the idea that the publisher is not required to render accounting, officially permitted, or otherwise, qualified services. If advice is necessary, legal or professional, a practiced individual in the profession should be ordered.

- From a Declaration of Principles which was accepted and approved equally by a Committee of the American Bar Association and a Committee of Publishers and Associations.

In no way is it legal to reproduce, duplicate, or transmit any part of this document in either electronic means or in printed format. Recording of this publication is strictly prohibited and any storage of this document is not allowed unless with written permission from the publisher. All rights reserved.

The information provided herein is stated to be truthful and consistent, in that any liability, in terms of inattention or otherwise, by any usage or abuse of any policies, processes, or directions contained within is the solitary and utter responsibility of the recipient reader. Under no circumstances will any legal responsibility or blame be held against the publisher for any reparation, damages, or monetary loss due to the information herein, either directly or indirectly.

Respective authors own all copyrights not held by the publisher.

The information herein is offered for informational

purposes solely, and is universal as so. The presentation of the information is without contract or any type of guarantee assurance.

The trademarks that are used are without any consent, and the publication of the trademark is without permission or backing by the trademark owner. All trademarks and brands within this book are for clarifying purposes only and are the owned by the owners themselves, not affiliated with this document.

Introduction

Low Carb High Fat recipes for personal enjoyment but also for family enjoyment. You will love them for sure for how easy it is to prepare them.

BREAKFAST

PINEAPPLE PANCAKES

Serves: **4**
Prep Time: **10** Minutes

Cook Time: **20** Minutes

Total Time: **30** Minutes

INGREDIENTS

- 1 cup whole wheat flour
- ¼ tsp baking soda
- ¼ tsp baking powder
- 1 cup pineapple
- 2 eggs
- 1 cup milk

DIRECTIONS

1. In a bowl combine all ingredients together and mix well
2. In a skillet heat olive oil

3. Pour ¼ of the batter and cook each pancake for 1-2 minutes per side
4. When ready remove from heat and serve

ALMOND PANCAKES

Serves: **4**
Prep Time: **10** Minutes
Cook Time: **30** Minutes
Total Time: **40** Minutes

INGREDIENTS

- 1 cup whole wheat flour
- ¼ tsp baking soda
- ¼ tsp baking powder
- 1 cup almonds
- 2 eggs
- 1 cup milk

DIRECTIONS

1. In a bowl combine all ingredients together and mix well
2. In a skillet heat olive oil
3. Pour ¼ of the batter and cook each pancake for 1-2 minutes per side

4. When ready remove from heat and serve

APPLE PANCAKES

Serves: **4**

Prep Time: **10** Minutes

Cook Time: **20** Minutes

Total Time: **30** Minutes

INGREDIENTS

- 1 cup whole wheat flour
- ¼ tsp baking soda
- ¼ tsp baking powder
- 1 cup mashed apple
- 2 eggs
- 1 cup milk

DIRECTIONS

1. In a bowl combine all ingredients together and mix well
2. In a skillet heat olive oil
3. Pour ¼ of the batter and cook each pancake for 1-2 minutes per side

4. When ready remove from heat and serve

STRAWBERRY PANCAKES

Serves: **4**

Prep Time: **10** Minutes

Cook Time: **20** Minutes

Total Time: **30** Minutes

INGREDIENTS

- 1 cup whole wheat flour
- ¼ tsp baking soda
- ¼ tsp baking powder
- 1 cup strawberries
- 2 eggs
- 1 cup milk

DIRECTIONS

1. In a bowl combine all ingredients together and mix well
2. In a skillet heat olive oil
3. Pour ¼ of the batter and cook each pancake for 1-2 minutes per side

4. When ready remove from heat and serve

PEAR PANCAKES

Serves: *4*
Prep Time: *10* Minutes
Cook Time: *30* Minutes
Total Time: *40* Minutes

INGREDIENTS

- 1 cup whole wheat flour
- ¼ tsp baking soda
- ¼ tsp baking powder
- 2 eggs
- 1 cup milk
- 1 cup mashed pear

DIRECTIONS

1. In a bowl combine all ingredients together and mix well
2. In a skillet heat olive oil
3. Pour ¼ of the batter and cook each pancake for 1-2 minutes per side

4. When ready remove from heat and serve

GINGERBREAD MUFFINS

Serves: **8-12**
Prep Time: **10** Minutes
Cook Time: **20** Minutes
Total Time: **30** Minutes

INGREDIENTS

- 2 eggs
- 1 tablespoon olive oil
- 1 cup milk
- 2 cups whole wheat flour
- 1 tsp baking soda
- ¼ tsp baking soda
- 1 tsp ginger
- 1 tsp cinnamon
- ¼ cup molasses

DIRECTIONS

1. In a bowl combine all dry ingredients
2. In another bowl combine all dry ingredients

3. Combine wet and dry ingredients together
4. Fold in ginger and mix well
5. Pour mixture into 8-12 prepared muffin cups, fill 2/3 of the cups
6. Bake for 18-20 minutes at 375 F
7. When ready remove from the oven and serve

CHERRIES MUFFINS

Serves: **8-12**
Prep Time: **10** Minutes
Cook Time: **20** Minutes
Total Time: **30** Minutes

INGREDIENTS

- 2 eggs
- 1 tablespoon olive oil
- 1 cup milk
- 2 cups whole wheat flour
- 1 tsp baking soda
- ¼ tsp baking soda
- 1 tsp cinnamon
- 1 cup mashed cherries

DIRECTIONS

1. In a bowl combine all dry ingredients
2. In another bowl combine all dry ingredients
3. Combine wet and dry ingredients together

4. Pour mixture into 8-12 prepared muffin cups, fill 2/3 of the cups
5. Bake for 18-20 minutes at 375 F
6. When ready remove from the oven and serve

BLUEBERRY MUFFINS

Serves: **8-12**

Prep Time: **10** Minutes

Cook Time: **20** Minutes

Total Time: **30** Minutes

INGREDIENTS

- 2 eggs
- 1 tablespoon olive oil
- 1 cup milk
- 2 cups whole wheat flour
- 1 tsp baking soda
- ¼ tsp baking soda
- 1 tsp cinnamon
- 1 cup blueberries

DIRECTIONS

1. In a bowl combine all dry ingredients
2. In another bowl combine all dry ingredients
3. Combine wet and dry ingredients together

4. Fold in blueberries and mix well
5. Pour mixture into 8-12 prepared muffin cups, fill 2/3 of the cups
6. Bake for 18-20 minutes at 375 F
7. When ready remove from the oven and serve

BERRIES MUFFINS

Serves: **8-12**
Prep Time: **10**   Minutes
Cook Time: **20**   Minutes
Total Time: **30**   Minutes

INGREDIENTS

- 2 eggs
- 1 tablespoon olive oil
- 1 cup milk
- 2 cups whole wheat flour
- 1 tsp baking soda
- ¼ tsp baking soda
- 1 tsp cinnamon
- 1 cup berries

DIRECTIONS

1. In a bowl combine all dry ingredients
2. In another bowl combine all dry ingredients
3. Combine wet and dry ingredients together

4. Pour mixture into 8-12 prepared muffin cups, fill 2/3 of the cups
5. Bake for 18-20 minutes at 375 F
6. When ready remove from the oven and serve

CHOCOLATE MUFFINS

Serves: **8-12**

Prep Time: **10** Minutes

Cook Time: **20** Minutes

Total Time: **30** Minutes

INGREDIENTS

- 2 eggs
- 1 tablespoon olive oil
- 1 cup milk
- 2 cups whole wheat flour
- 1 tsp baking soda
- ¼ tsp baking soda
- 1 tsp cinnamon
- 1 cup chocolate chips

DIRECTIONS

1. **In a bowl combine all dry ingredients**
2. **In another bowl combine all dry ingredients**
3. **Combine wet and dry ingredients together**

4. Fold in chocolate chips and mix well
5. Pour mixture into 8-12 prepared muffin cups, fill 2/3 of the cups
6. Bake for 18-20 minutes at 375 F
7. When ready remove from the oven and serve

RASPBERRIES MUFFINS

Serves: **8-12**
Prep Time: **10** Minutes
Cook Time: **20** Minutes
Total Time: **30** Minutes

INGREDIENTS

- 2 eggs
- 1 tablespoon olive oil
- 1 cup milk
- 2 cups whole wheat flour
- 1 tsp baking soda
- ¼ tsp baking soda
- 1 tsp cinnamon
- 1 cup raspberries

DIRECTIONS

1. In a bowl combine all dry ingredients
2. In another bowl combine all dry ingredients
3. Combine wet and dry ingredients together

4. Pour mixture into 8-12 prepared muffin cups, fill 2/3 of the cups
5. Bake for 18-20 minutes at 375 F
6. When ready remove from the oven and serve

LETTUCE OMELETTE

Serves: *1*
Prep Time: *5* Minutes
Cook Time: *10* Minutes
Total Time: *15* Minutes

INGREDIENTS

- 2 eggs
- ¼ tsp salt
- ¼ tsp black pepper
- 1 tablespoon olive oil
- ¼ cup cheese
- ¼ tsp basil
- 1 bunch lettuce

DIRECTIONS

1. In a bowl combine all ingredients together and mix well
2. In a skillet heat olive oil and pour the egg mixture

3. Cook for 1-2 minutes per side
4. When ready remove omelette from the skillet and serve

ZUCCHINI OMELETTE

Serves: **1**
Prep Time: **5** Minutes
Cook Time: **10** Minutes
Total Time: **15** Minutes

INGREDIENTS

- 2 eggs
- ¼ tsp salt
- ¼ tsp black pepper
- 1 tablespoon olive oil
- ¼ cup cheese
- ¼ tsp basil
- 1 cup zucchini

DIRECTIONS

1. In a bowl combine all ingredients together and mix well
2. In a skillet heat olive oil and pour the egg mixture

3. Cook for 1-2 minutes per side
4. When ready remove omelette from the skillet and serve

JICAMA OMELETTE

Serves: *1*
Prep Time: *5* Minutes
Cook Time: *10* Minutes
Total Time: *15* Minutes

INGREDIENTS

- 2 eggs
- ¼ tsp salt
- ¼ tsp black pepper
- 1 tablespoon olive oil
- ¼ cup cheese
- ¼ tsp basil
- ½ cup jicama
- 1 cup red onion

DIRECTIONS

1. **In a bowl combine all ingredients together and mix well**

2. In a skillet heat olive oil and pour the egg mixture
3. Cook for 1-2 minutes per side
4. When ready remove omelette from the skillet and serve

MUSHROOM OMELETTE

Serves: **1**
Prep Time: **5** Minutes
Cook Time: **10** Minutes
Total Time: **15** Minutes

INGREDIENTS

- 2 eggs
- ¼ tsp salt
- ¼ tsp black pepper
- 1 tablespoon olive oil
- ¼ cup cheese
- ¼ tsp basil
- 1 cup mushrooms

DIRECTIONS

1. In a bowl combine all ingredients together and mix well
2. In a skillet heat olive oil and pour the egg mixture

3. Cook for 1-2 minutes per side
4. When ready remove omelette from the skillet and serve

BASIL OMELETTE

Serves: **1**
Prep Time: **5** Minutes
Cook Time: **10** Minutes
Total Time: **15** Minutes

INGREDIENTS

- 2 eggs
- ¼ tsp salt
- ¼ tsp black pepper
- 1 tablespoon olive oil
- ¼ cup cheese
- ¼ tsp basil
- 1 cup tomatoes

DIRECTIONS

1. In a bowl combine all ingredients together and mix well
2. In a skillet heat olive oil and pour the egg mixture

3. Cook for 1-2 minutes per side
4. When ready remove omelette from the skillet and serve

HASH BROWN EGG NESTS

Serves: **4**

Prep Time: **10** Minutes

Cook Time: **30** Minutes

Total Time: **40** Minutes

INGREDIENTS

- 12 oz. hash browns
- 1 cup cheddar cheese
- 1 tablespoon olive oil
- 6 eggs
- 2-3 slices bacon
- 1 tablespoon parsley

DIRECTIONS

1. In a bowl combine hash browns, olive oil and set aside
2. Pour the mixture into a prepare baking dish and top with cheese
3. Bake at 400 F for 10-12 minutes or until cheese has melted

4. Beat the eggs with bacon and parsley
5. Pour egg mixture over and bake for another 12-15 minutes at 375 F
6. When ready remove from the oven and serve

BREAKFAST BARS

Serves: **6-8**
Prep Time: **10**   Minutes
Cook Time: **60**   Minutes
Total Time: **70**   Minutes

INGREDIENTS

- ½ cup honey
- ½ cup peanut butter
- 1 tsp vanilla extract
- 1 cup rice cereal
- 1 cup oats
- 1 tablespoon flax seed
- 1 tablespoon raisins

DIRECTIONS

1. **In a bowl combine all ingredients together**
2. **Add honey, peanut butter and combine until everything is sticky**

3. Pour mixture into a pan and refrigerate for 30-60 minutes
4. When ready cut into bars and serve

MORNING GRANOLA

Serves: **4**

Prep Time: **10** Minutes

Cook Time: **30** Minutes

Total Time: **40** Minutes

INGREDIENTS

- 2 cups oats
- 1 cup almonds
- ¼ cup coconut flakes
- ¼ tsp cinnamon
- ¼ cup maple syrup
- 1 tablespoon brown sugar
- 1 cup raisins

DIRECTIONS

1. In a bowl combine all ingredients together
2. Add maple syrup and mix well
3. Spread mixture into a pan and bake for 30 minutes at 325 F

4. When ready remove from the oven and serve

STREUSEL SCONES

Serves: **4**

Prep Time: **10** Minutes

Cook Time: **30** Minutes

Total Time: **40** Minutes

INGREDIENTS

- 2 cups almond flour
- ¼ cup brown sugar
- 1 tsp baking powder
- ¼ tsp salt
- 4 tablespoons olive oil
- 1 cup blueberries
- 1 egg
- 1 tsp vanilla extract
- 1 cup almond milk

DIRECTIONS

1. **In a bowl combine flour, sugar, baking powder and place aside**

2. In another bowl whisk the egg with vanilla extract and pour the flour mixture into the egg mixture
3. Add blueberries and mix well
4. Place everything in the oven and bake at 375 F until golden brown
5. When ready serve streusel topping

LUNCH

PUMPKIN FRITATTA

Serves: **2**
Prep Time: **10** Minutes
Cook Time: **20** Minutes
Total Time: **30** Minutes

INGREDIENTS

- ½ lb. pumpkin puree
- 1 tablespoon olive oil
- ½ red onion
- ¼ tsp salt
- 2 oz. cheddar cheese
- 1 garlic clove
- ¼ tsp dill

DIRECTIONS

1. **In a bowl whisk eggs with salt and cheese**

2. In a frying pan heat olive oil and pour egg mixture
3. Add remaining ingredients and mix well
4. Serve when ready

SPINACH FRITATTA

Serves: **2**
Prep Time: **10** Minutes
Cook Time: **20** Minutes
Total Time: **30** Minutes

INGREDIENTS

- ½ lb. spinach
- 1 tablespoon olive oil
- ½ red onion
- ¼ tsp salt
- 2 oz. cheddar cheese
- 1 garlic clove
- ¼ tsp dill

DIRECTIONS

1. In a bowl whisk eggs with salt and cheese
2. In a frying pan heat olive oil and pour egg mixture
3. Add remaining ingredients and mix well

4. Serve when ready

KALE FRITATTA

Serves: **2**

Prep Time: **10** Minutes

Cook Time: **20** Minutes

Total Time: **30** Minutes

INGREDIENTS

- 1 cup kale
- 1 tablespoon olive oil
- ½ red onion
- ¼ tsp salt
- 2 oz. cheddar cheese
- 1 garlic clove
- ¼ tsp dill

DIRECTIONS

1. In a skillet sauté kale until tender
2. In a bowl whisk eggs with salt and cheese
3. In a frying pan heat olive oil and pour egg mixture

4. Add remaining ingredients and mix well
5. When ready serve with sautéed kale

SNOW PEAS FRITATTA

Serves: **2**
Prep Time: **10** Minutes
Cook Time: **20** Minutes
Total Time: **30** Minutes

INGREDIENTS

- ½ cup snow peas
- 1 tablespoon olive oil
- ½ red onion
- ¼ tsp salt
- 2 oz. parmesan cheese
- 1 garlic clove
- ¼ tsp dill

DIRECTIONS

1. In a bowl whisk eggs with salt and parmesan cheese
2. In a frying pan heat olive oil and pour egg mixture

3. Add remaining ingredients and mix well
4. Serve when ready

BROCCOLI FRITATTA

Serves: **2**

Prep Time: **10** Minutes

Cook Time: **20** Minutes

Total Time: **30** Minutes

INGREDIENTS

- 1 cup broccoli
- 1 tablespoon olive oil
- ½ red onion
- ¼ tsp salt
- 2 oz. cheddar cheese
- 1 garlic clove
- ¼ tsp dill

DIRECTIONS

1. In a skillet sauté broccoli until tender
2. In a bowl whisk eggs with salt and cheese
3. In a frying pan heat olive oil and pour egg mixture

4. Add remaining ingredients and mix well
5. When ready serve with sautéed broccoli

SALMON WITH HERB SAUCE

Serves: 2
Prep Time: 10 Minutes
Cook Time: 35 Minutes
Total Time: 45 Minutes

INGREDIENTS

- 2 salmon fillets
- 2 tablespoons butter
- 1 tablespoon flour
- 1 tsp tarragon
- 5-6 sage leaves
- 1 tablespoon parsley

DIRECTIONS

1. In a dish combine all ingredients together except the salmon fillets
2. Spread the mixture over the salmon fillet and rub the fish with it
3. Place the salmon in the oven at 325 F for 30-35 minutes

4. When ready remove from the oven and serve

GLAZED PORK CHOPS

Serves: **2**

Prep Time: **10** Minutes

Cook Time: **20** Minutes

Total Time: **30** Minutes

INGREDIENTS

- ½ cup dark rum
- ¼ cup maple syrup
- ¼ cup olive oil
- 2 pork chops
- marinade

DIRECTIONS

1. In a bowl prepare the marinade for the pork chops and set aside
2. Add the pork chops to marinade, refrigerate for 50-60 minutes
3. Place the rum, maple syrup and olive oil in a saucepan and bring to a boil

4. Place the pork chops in a skillet and cook on low heat
5. Pour glaze from the saucepan over the pork chops and cook until pork chops are cooked
6. When ready transfer to a plate and serve

VEGGIES PIZZA

Serves: **1**

Prep Time: **10** Minutes

Cook Time: **15** Minutes

Total Time: **25** Minutes

INGREDIENTS

- ½ cup zucchini
- ½ cup mushrooms
- ¼ cup black olives
- 1 pizza dough
- ½ cup tomato sauce
- ¼ cup parmesan cheese
- 1 cup mozzarella cheese
- Olive oil

DIRECTIONS

1. In a bowl combine all vegetables and drizzle olive oil and salt over vegetables

2. On a pizza dough spread tomato sauce, vegetables and top with mozzarella and parmesan cheese
3. Bake at 400 F for 12-15 minutes
4. When ready remove from the oven and serve

LIVER AND MASHED VEGETABLES

Serves: **4**

Prep Time: **20** Minutes

Cook Time: **40** Minutes

Total Time: **60** Minutes

INGREDIENTS

- 3 tsp rapeseed oil
- 350g sweet potato
- 150g parsnip
- 320g green beans
- 350g swede
- 3 cloves garlic
- 15 g flour
- 4 onions
- 1 pack liver
- 1 cube lamb stock
- Black pepper

DIRECTIONS

1. Cook the onions in hot oil for about 20 minutes
2. Coat the liver with flour and pepper and cook in a pan until brown
3. Add the garlic to the onions and stir in 2 tsp of flour
4. Dissolve the stock cube in 450 ml water, then pour over the onions and bring to a boil
5. Add the liver and cook for 5 more minutes
6. Boil the vegetables covered for about 15 minutes
7. Mash the potato, parsnip and swede together
8. Serve the liver with the mashed vegetables

LEMON CHICKEN

Serves: **4**
Prep Time: **10** Minutes
Cook Time: **20** Minutes
Total Time: **30** Minutes

INGREDIENTS

- 3 tsp garlic
- 5 tbs lemon juice
- 4 tbs butter
- 4 chicken breasts
- ½ cup chicken broth
- 1 ½ tbs honey
- 2 tsp seasoning
- Salt
- Pepper

DIRECTIONS

1. Cook the chicken in melted butter until golden on both sides

2. Mix the lemon juice, chicken broth, garlic, honey, salt, pepper, and seasoning in a bowl
3. Place the chicken on a baking sheet and pour the sauce over
4. Bake in the preheated oven for at least 20 minutes at 350F spooning the sauce over the chicken every 5 minutes
5. Serve with lemon slices

CALIFORNIA SALAD

Serves: **2**
Prep Time: **5** Minutes
Cook Time: **5** Minutes
Total Time: **10** Minutes

INGREDIENTS

- 2-3 cups broccoli slaw
- 1-2 bunches green onion
- 1 tablespoon olive oil
- 1 package cooked noodles
- salad dressing

DIRECTIONS

1. **In a bowl mix all ingredients and mix well**
2. **Serve with dressing**

QUINOA SALAD

Serves: 2
Prep Time: 5 Minutes
Cook Time: 5 Minutes
Total Time: 10 Minutes

INGREDIENTS

- 1 cup cooked quinoa
- 1 handful of spinach leaves
- 1 pear
- ¼ cup black beans
- ¼ cup bell pepper
- ¼ cup cucumber
- ¼ cup zucchini

DIRECTIONS

1. In a bowl mix all ingredients and mix well
2. Serve with dressing

PANZANELLA SALAD

Serves: **2**

Prep Time: **5** Minutes

Cook Time: **5** Minutes

Total Time: **10** Minutes

INGREDIENTS

- 1 lb. tomatoes
- 1 tsp salt
- 1 lb. ciabatta
- 2 tablespoons olive oil
- 2-3 shallots
- 2 garlic cloves
- 1 tsp mustard
- ¼ cup basil leaves

DIRECTIONS

1. In a bowl mix all ingredients and mix well
2. Serve with dressing

BASIL SALAD

Serves: **2**
Prep Time: **5** Minutes
Cook Time: **5** Minutes
Total Time: **10** Minutes

INGREDIENTS

- 1 cup olive oil
- ¼ cup basil
- 1 lb. mozzarella
- 1-pint cherry
- 2 tablespoons balsamic vinegar

DIRECTIONS

1. **In a bowl mix all ingredients and mix well**
2. **Serve with dressing**

TOMATO SALAD

Serves: **2**
Prep Time: **5** Minutes
Cook Time: **5** Minutes
Total Time: **10** Minutes

INGREDIENTS

- 1 lb. tomatoes
- 1 tsp salt
- 1 shallot
- 1 red onion
- 1 cup salad dressing
- 1 cup olives
- 1 cucumber
- ½ cup feta cheese

DIRECTIONS

1. In a bowl mix all ingredients and mix well
2. Serve with dressing

POTATO SALAD

Serves: 2
Prep Time: 5 Minutes
Cook Time: 5 Minutes
Total Time: 10 Minutes

INGREDIENTS

- 1 lb. cooked sweet potatoes
- 2 tablespoons olive oil
- 1 tsp mustard
- 1 red onion
- 3 tablespoons chives
- 1 cup olives
- 1 cup pickles

DIRECTIONS

1. In a bowl mix all ingredients and mix well
2. Serve with dressing

HAWAIIAN SALAD

Serves: **2**

Prep Time: **5** Minutes

Cook Time: **5** Minutes

Total Time: **10** Minutes

INGREDIENTS

- 1 tsp hijiki
- 8 oz. tuna
- 2 oz. red onion
- 1 scallion
- 1 tsp sesame seeds
- 2 tsp soy sauce
- 2 tsp sesame oil
- 1/4 cup steamed rice

DIRECTIONS

1. **In a bowl mix all ingredients and mix well**
2. **Serve with dressing**

COLESLAW

Serves: **2**

Prep Time: **5** Minutes

Cook Time: **5** Minutes

Total Time: **10** Minutes

INGREDIENTS

- 1 cabbage
- 1 red onion
- 1 carrot
- ¼ cup leaves
- 1 cup coleslaw dressing

DIRECTIONS

1. In a bowl mix all ingredients and mix well
2. Serve with dressing

KALE SALAD

Serves: **2**
Prep Time: **5** Minutes
Cook Time: **5** Minutes
Total Time: **10** Minutes

INGREDIENTS

- 1 lb. kale
- 4 tablespoons olive oil
- 5-6 anchovy fillets
- 1 clove garlic
- 1 red onion
- 1 cup Caesar salad dressing

DIRECTIONS

1. **In a bowl mix all ingredients and mix well**
2. **Serve with dressing**

ICEBERG WEDGE SALAD

Serves: **2**
Prep Time: **5** Minutes
Cook Time: **5** Minutes
Total Time: **10** Minutes

INGREDIENTS

- 2 tomatoes
- 1 red onion
- 4-5 oz. bacon
- 3-4 oz. bread crumbs
- 1 head iceberg lettuce
- 1 tsp black pepper
- 1 cup salad dressing

DIRECTIONS

1. **In a bowl mix all ingredients and mix well**
2. **Serve with dressing**

DINNER

SIMPLE PIZZA RECIPE

Serves: **6-8**
Prep Time: **10** Minutes
Cook Time: **15** Minutes
Total Time: **25** Minutes

INGREDIENTS

- 1 pizza crust
- ½ cup tomato sauce
- ¼ black pepper
- 1 cup pepperoni slices
- 1 cup mozzarella cheese
- 1 cup olives

DIRECTIONS

1. Spread tomato sauce on the pizza crust
2. Place all the toppings on the pizza crust
3. Bake the pizza at 425 F for 12-15 minutes

4. When ready remove pizza from the oven and serve

ZUCCHINI PIZZA

Serves: **6-8**
Prep Time: **10** Minutes
Cook Time: **15** Minutes
Total Time: **25** Minutes

INGREDIENTS

- 1 pizza crust
- ½ cup tomato sauce
- ¼ black pepper
- 1 cup zucchini slices
- 1 cup mozzarella cheese
- 1 cup olives

DIRECTIONS

1. Spread tomato sauce on the pizza crust
2. Place all the toppings on the pizza crust
3. Bake the pizza at 425 F for 12-15 minutes
4. When ready remove pizza from the oven and serve

CAULIFLOWER RECIPE

Serves: **6-8**
Prep Time: **10** Minutes
Cook Time: **15** Minutes
Total Time: **25** Minutes

INGREDIENTS

- 1 pizza crust
- ½ cup tomato sauce
- ¼ black pepper
- 1 cup cauliflower
- 1 cup mozzarella cheese
- 1 cup olives

DIRECTIONS

1. Spread tomato sauce on the pizza crust
2. Place all the toppings on the pizza crust
3. Bake the pizza at 425 F for 12-15 minutes
4. When ready remove pizza from the oven and serve

BROCCOLI RECIPE

Serves: **6-8**

Prep Time: **10** Minutes

Cook Time: **15** Minutes

Total Time: **25** Minutes

INGREDIENTS

- 1 pizza crust
- ½ cup tomato sauce
- ¼ black pepper
- 1 cup broccoli
- 1 cup mozzarella cheese
- 1 cup olives

DIRECTIONS

1. Spread tomato sauce on the pizza crust
2. Place all the toppings on the pizza crust
3. Bake the pizza at 425 F for 12-15 minutes
4. When ready remove pizza from the oven and serve

TOMATOES & HAM PIZZA

Serves: **6-8**
Prep Time: **10** Minutes
Cook Time: **15** Minutes
Total Time: **25** Minutes

INGREDIENTS

- 1 pizza crust
- ½ cup tomato sauce
- ¼ black pepper
- 1 cup pepperoni slices
- 1 cup tomatoes
- 6-8 ham slices
- 1 cup mozzarella cheese
- 1 cup olives

DIRECTIONS

1. Spread tomato sauce on the pizza crust
2. Place all the toppings on the pizza crust
3. Bake the pizza at 425 F for 12-15 minutes

4. When ready remove pizza from the oven and serve

LEEK SOUP

Serves: **4**

Prep Time: **10** Minutes

Cook Time: **20** Minutes

Total Time: **30** Minutes

INGREDIENTS

- 1 tablespoon olive oil
- 1 lb. leeks
- ¼ red onion
- ½ cup all-purpose flour
- ¼ tsp salt
- ¼ tsp pepper
- 1 can vegetable broth
- 1 cup heavy cream

DIRECTIONS

1. In a saucepan heat olive oil and sauté onion until tender

2. Add remaining ingredients to the saucepan and bring to a boil
3. When all the vegetables are tender transfer to a blender and blend until smooth
4. Pour soup into bowls, garnish with parsley and serve

ZUCCHINI SOUP

Serves: **4**
Prep Time: **10** Minutes
Cook Time: **20** Minutes
Total Time: **30** Minutes

INGREDIENTS

- 1 tablespoon olive oil
- 1 lb. zucchini
- ¼ red onion
- ½ cup all-purpose flour
- ¼ tsp salt
- ¼ tsp pepper
- 1 can vegetable broth
- 1 cup heavy cream

DIRECTIONS

1. In a saucepan heat olive oil and sauté onion until tender

2. Add remaining ingredients to the saucepan and bring to a boil
3. When all the vegetables are tender transfer to a blender and blend until smooth
4. Pour soup into bowls, garnish with parsley and serve

OKRA SOUP

Serves: **4**

Prep Time: **10** Minutes

Cook Time: **20** Minutes

Total Time: **30** Minutes

INGREDIENTS

- 1 tablespoon olive oil
- 1 lb. okra
- ¼ red onion
- ½ cup all-purpose flour
- ¼ tsp salt
- ¼ tsp pepper
- 1 can vegetable broth
- 1 cup heavy cream

DIRECTIONS

1. **In a saucepan heat olive oil and sauté onion until tender**

2. Add remaining ingredients to the saucepan and bring to a boil
3. When all the vegetables are tender transfer to a blender and blend until smooth
4. Pour soup into bowls, garnish with parsley and serve

RED BELL PEPPER SOUP

Serves: **4**
Prep Time: **10** Minutes
Cook Time: **20** Minutes
Total Time: **30** Minutes

INGREDIENTS

- 1 tablespoon olive oil
- 1 lb. red bell pepper
- ¼ red onion
- ½ cup all-purpose flour
- ¼ tsp salt
- ¼ tsp pepper
- 1 can vegetable broth
- 1 cup heavy cream

DIRECTIONS

1. In a saucepan heat olive oil and sauté onion until tender

2. Add remaining ingredients to the saucepan and bring to a boil
3. When all the vegetables are tender transfer to a blender and blend until smooth
4. Pour soup into bowls, garnish with parsley and serve

POTATO SOUP

Serves: **4**

Prep Time: **10** Minutes

Cook Time: **20** Minutes

Total Time: **30** Minutes

INGREDIENTS

- 1 tablespoon olive oil
- 1 lb. mushrooms
- ¼ red onion
- ½ cup all-purpose flour
- ¼ tsp salt
- ¼ tsp pepper
- 1 can vegetable broth
- 1 cup heavy cream

DIRECTIONS

1. **In a saucepan heat olive oil and sauté potatoes until tender**

2. Add remaining ingredients to the saucepan and bring to a boil
3. When all the vegetables are tender transfer to a blender and blend until smooth
4. Pour soup into bowls, garnish with parsley and serve

SMOOTHIES

PINK SMOOTHIE

Serves: **1**
Prep Time: **5** Minutes
Cook Time: **5** Minutes
Total Time: **10** Minutes

INGREDIENTS

- 2 bananas
- ½ cup dragon fruit
- 1 tsp coconut flakes
- 1 tsp coconut flakes
- 1 cup coconut water

DIRECTIONS

1. In a blender place all ingredients and blend until smooth
2. Pour smoothie in a glass and serve

APPLE BANANA SMOOTHIE

Serves: **1**
Prep Time: **5** Minutes
Cook Time: **5** Minutes
Total Time: **10** Minutes

INGREDIENTS

- 1 banana
- 1 apple
- 3 tablespoons peanut butter
- ¼ cup almonds
- 1 cup ice

DIRECTIONS

1. **In a blender place all ingredients and blend until smooth**
2. **Pour smoothie in a glass and serve**

CARDAMOM SMOOTHIE

Serves: **1**
Prep Time: **5** Minutes
Cook Time: **5** Minutes
Total Time: **10** Minutes

INGREDIENTS

- 1 beetroot
- 1 cup coconut milk
- 1 banana
- 2 cardamom seeds
- 1 cup ice
- 1 tsp vanilla extract
- 1 tsp lemon juice

DIRECTIONS

1. **In a blender place all ingredients and blend until smooth**
2. **Pour smoothie in a glass and serve**

VEGAN SMOOTHIE

Serves: *1*
Prep Time: *5* Minutes
Cook Time: *5* Minutes
Total Time: *10* Minutes

INGREDIENTS

- 1 banana
- 2 tablespoons oats
- 2 tsp nut butter
- 2 tsp pumpkin puree
- 1 cup soy milk

DIRECTIONS

1. In a blender place all ingredients and blend until smooth
2. Pour smoothie in a glass and serve

BLACKBERRY SMOOTHIE

Serves: *1*
Prep Time: *5* Minutes
Cook Time: *5* Minutes
Total Time: *10* Minutes

INGREDIENTS

- 1 lb. berries
- 1 apple
- 1 cup coconut milk
- ¼ cup vanilla yogurt
- 2 oz. oats

DIRECTIONS

1. **In a blender place all ingredients and blend until smooth**
2. **Pour smoothie in a glass and serve**

STRAWBERRY SMOOTHIE

Serves: *1*

Prep Time: *5* Minutes

Cook Time: *5* Minutes

Total Time: *10* Minutes

INGREDIENTS

- 1 lb. strawberries
- ½ cup vanilla yogurt
- 1 tsp brown sugar
- 1 cup ice

DIRECTIONS

1. **In a blender place all ingredients and blend until smooth**
2. **Pour smoothie in a glass and serve**

MANGO SMOOTHIE

Serves: **1**
Prep Time: **5** Minutes
Cook Time: **5** Minutes
Total Time: **10** Minutes

INGREDIENTS

- 1 mango
- 1 banana
- 1 cup vanilla yogurt
- 1 cup ice

DIRECTIONS

1. In a blender place all ingredients and blend until smooth
2. Pour smoothie in a glass and serve

BANANA SMOOTHIE

Serves: **1**

Prep Time: **5** Minutes

Cook Time: **5** Minutes

Total Time: **10** Minutes

INGREDIENTS

- 1 cup vanilla yogurt
- 1 banana
- 1 cup skimmed milk
- 1 tsp cinnamon

DIRECTIONS

1. **In a blender place all ingredients and blend until smooth**
2. **Pour smoothie in a glass and serve**

SUMMER SMOOTHIE

Serves: **1**

Prep Time: **5** Minutes

Cook Time: **5** Minutes

Total Time: **10** Minutes

INGREDIENTS

- 5 oz. blueberries
- 1 banana
- 1 tsp vanilla yogurt
- 1 cup milk
- 1 tsp brown sugar
- 1 cup ice

DIRECTIONS

1. In a blender place all ingredients and blend until smooth
2. Pour smoothie in a glass and serve

DETOX SMOOTHIE

Serves: **1**
Prep Time: **5** Minutes
Cook Time: **5** Minutes
Total Time: **10** Minutes

INGREDIENTS

- 2 oz. kale
- 2 oz. spinach
- 2 oz. skimmed milk
- 1 banana
- 1 kiwi
- 3 oz. pineapple
- 1 apple

DIRECTIONS

1. **In a blender place all ingredients and blend until smooth**
2. **Pour smoothie in a glass and serve**

THANK YOU FOR READING THIS BOOK!

CPSIA information can be obtained
at www.ICGtesting.com
Printed in the USA
FSHW011928230121
77942FS

9 781706 033387